Blood Sugar Tracker

~weekly set up to track daily readings
~ includes images to color for your enjoyme

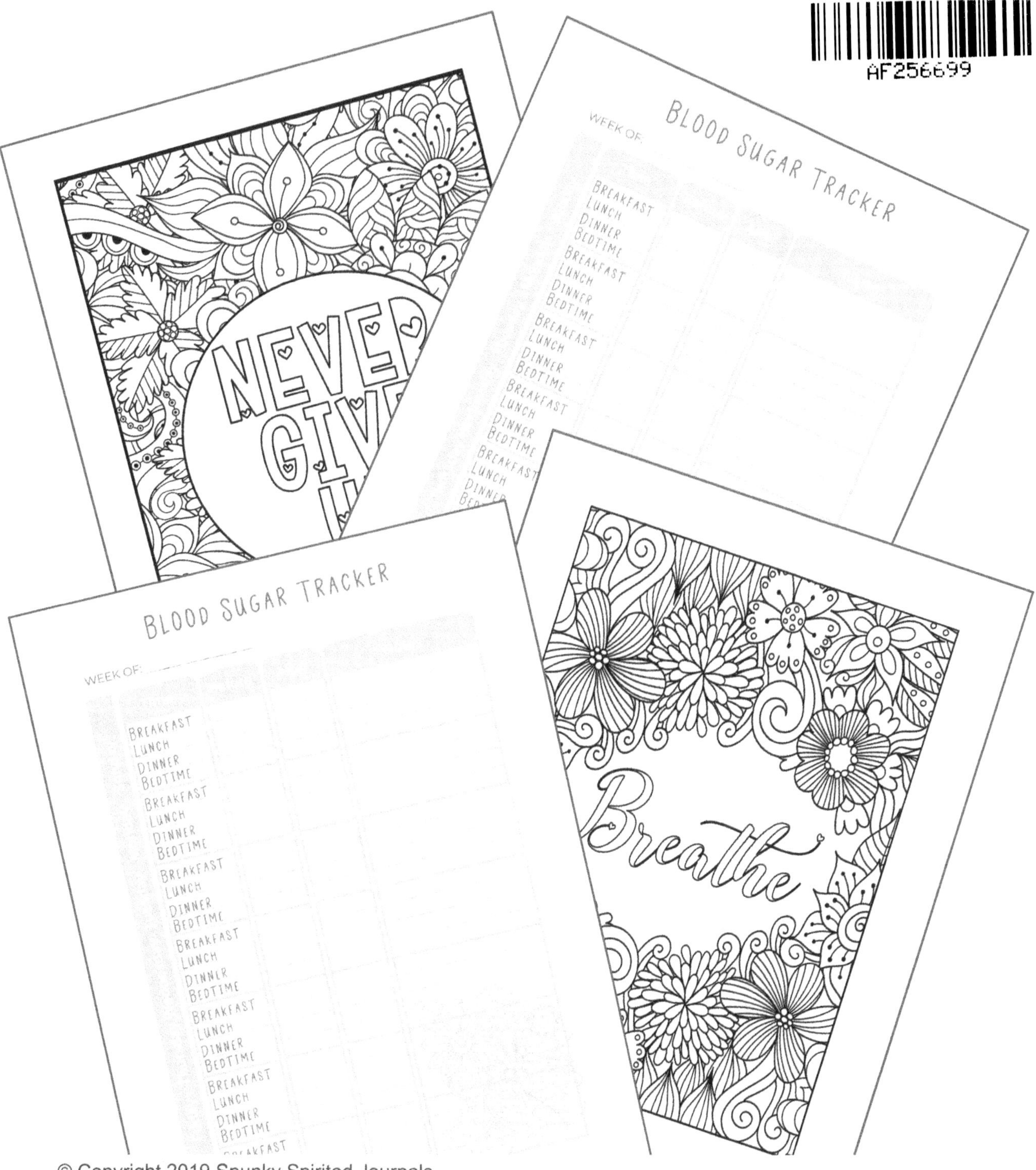

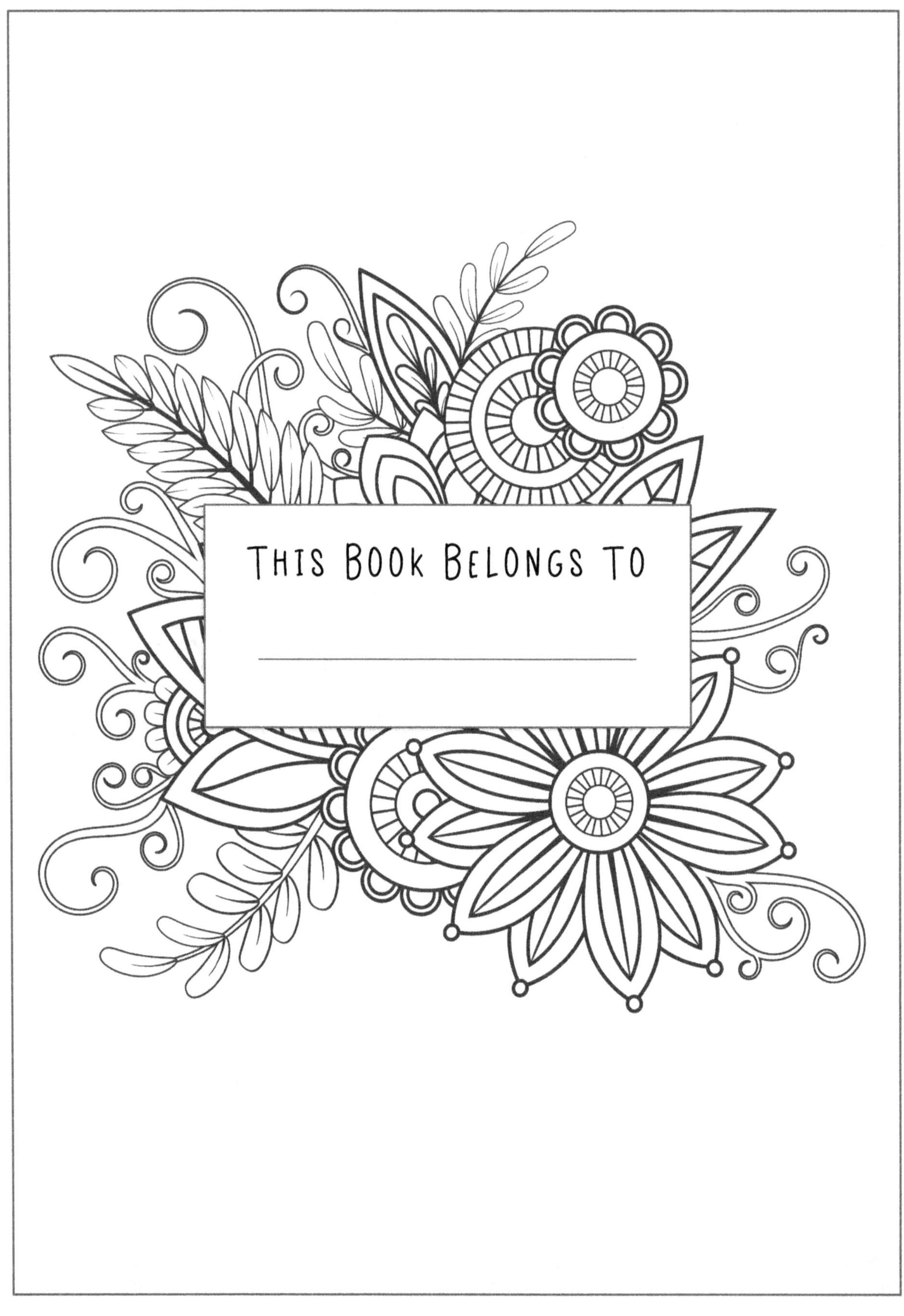

THIS BOOK BELONGS TO

Blood Sugar Tracker

WEEK OF: _____________________

	Time	Before	After	Notes
	Breakfast			
	Lunch			
	Dinner			
	Bedtime			
	Breakfast			
	Lunch			
	Dinner			
	Bedtime			
	Breakfast			
	Lunch			
	Dinner			
	Bedtime			
	Breakfast			
	Lunch			
	Dinner			
	Bedtime			
	Breakfast			
	Lunch			
	Dinner			
	Bedtime			
	Breakfast			
	Lunch			
	Dinner			
	Bedtime			
	Breakfast			
	Lunch			
	Dinner			
	Bedtime			

Blood Sugar Tracker

WEEK OF: ________________

	Time	Before	After	Notes
Sunday	Breakfast Lunch Dinner Bedtime			
Monday	Breakfast Lunch Dinner Bedtime			
Tuesday	Breakfast Lunch Dinner Bedtime			
Wednesday	Breakfast Lunch Dinner Bedtime			
Thursday	Breakfast Lunch Dinner Bedtime			
Friday	Breakfast Lunch Dinner Bedtime			
Saturday	Breakfast Lunch Dinner Bedtime			

Blood Sugar Tracker

WEEK OF: _______________________

	Time	Before	After	Notes
Sunday	Breakfast Lunch Dinner Bedtime			
Monday	Breakfast Lunch Dinner Bedtime			
Tuesday	Breakfast Lunch Dinner Bedtime			
Wednesday	Breakfast Lunch Dinner Bedtime			
Thursday	Breakfast Lunch Dinner Bedtime			
Friday	Breakfast Lunch Dinner Bedtime			
Saturday	Breakfast Lunch Dinner Bedtime			

Blood Sugar Tracker

WEEK OF: _______________

	Time	Before	After	Notes
Sunday	Breakfast Lunch Dinner Bedtime			
Monday	Breakfast Lunch Dinner Bedtime			
Tuesday	Breakfast Lunch Dinner Bedtime			
Wednesday	Breakfast Lunch Dinner Bedtime			
Thursday	Breakfast Lunch Dinner Bedtime			
Friday	Breakfast Lunch Dinner Bedtime			
Saturday	Breakfast Lunch Dinner Bedtime			

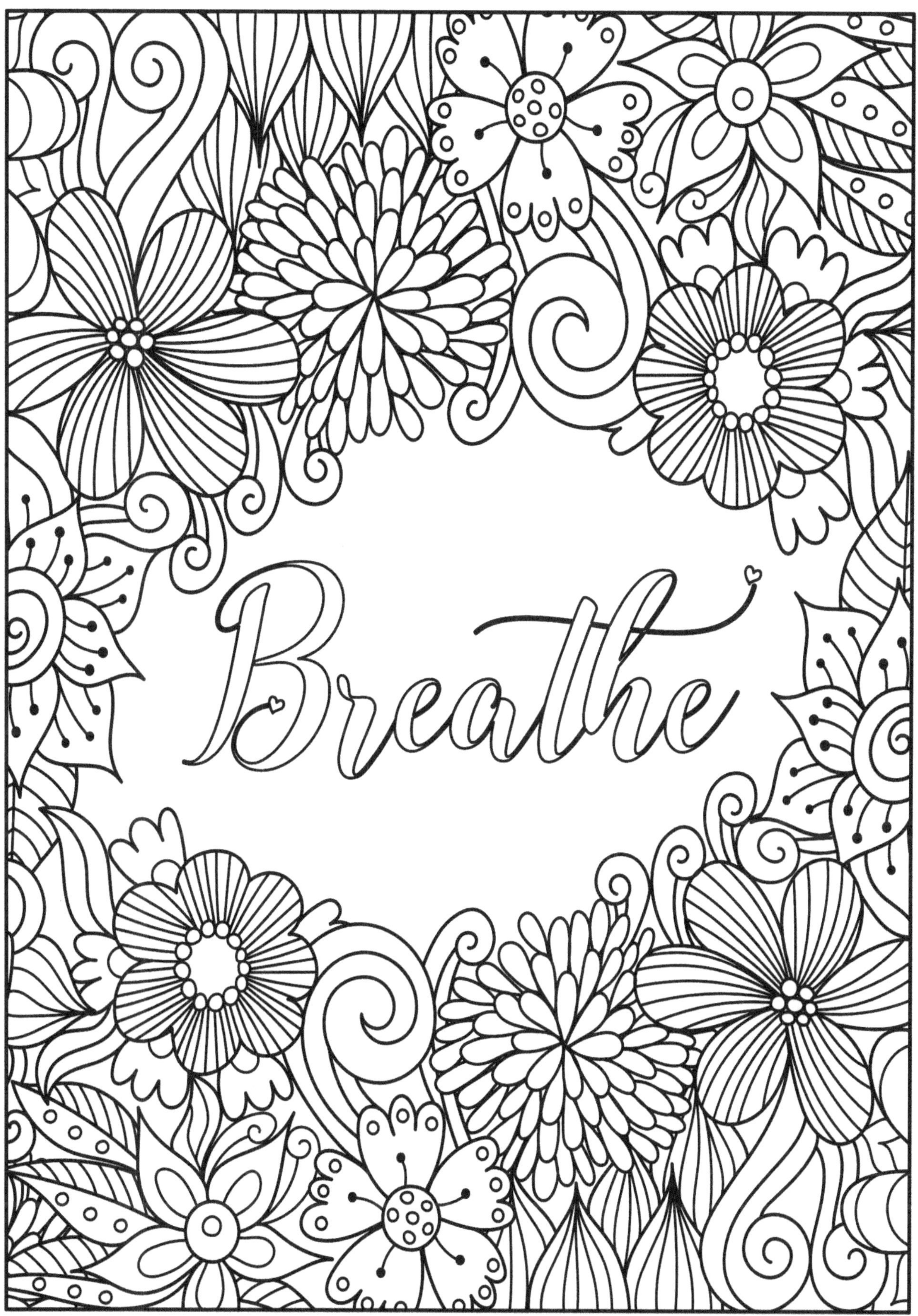
Breathe

Blood Sugar Tracker

WEEK OF: _______________________

Time	Before	After	Notes
Breakfast			
Lunch			
Dinner			
Bedtime			
Breakfast			
Lunch			
Dinner			
Bedtime			
Breakfast			
Lunch			
Dinner			
Bedtime			
Breakfast			
Lunch			
Dinner			
Bedtime			
Breakfast			
Lunch			
Dinner			
Bedtime			
Breakfast			
Lunch			
Dinner			
Bedtime			
Breakfast			
Lunch			
Dinner			
Bedtime			

Blood Sugar Tracker

WEEK OF: _________________

	Time	Before	After	Notes
Sunday	Breakfast			
	Lunch			
	Dinner			
	Bedtime			
Monday	Breakfast			
	Lunch			
	Dinner			
	Bedtime			
Tuesday	Breakfast			
	Lunch			
	Dinner			
	Bedtime			
Wednesday	Breakfast			
	Lunch			
	Dinner			
	Bedtime			
Thursday	Breakfast			
	Lunch			
	Dinner			
	Bedtime			
Friday	Breakfast			
	Lunch			
	Dinner			
	Bedtime			
Saturday	Breakfast			
	Lunch			
	Dinner			
	Bedtime			

Blood Sugar Tracker

WEEK OF: _________________

Time	Before	After	Notes
Breakfast			
Lunch			
Dinner			
Bedtime			
Breakfast			
Lunch			
Dinner			
Bedtime			
Breakfast			
Lunch			
Dinner			
Bedtime			
Breakfast			
Lunch			
Dinner			
Bedtime			
Breakfast			
Lunch			
Dinner			
Bedtime			
Breakfast			
Lunch			
Dinner			
Bedtime			
Breakfast			
Lunch			
Dinner			
Bedtime			

Blood Sugar Tracker

WEEK OF: _________________

	Time	Before	After	Notes
Sunday	Breakfast			
	Lunch			
	Dinner			
	Bedtime			
Monday	Breakfast			
	Lunch			
	Dinner			
	Bedtime			
Tuesday	Breakfast			
	Lunch			
	Dinner			
	Bedtime			
Wednesday	Breakfast			
	Lunch			
	Dinner			
	Bedtime			
Thursday	Breakfast			
	Lunch			
	Dinner			
	Bedtime			
Friday	Breakfast			
	Lunch			
	Dinner			
	Bedtime			
Saturday	Breakfast			
	Lunch			
	Dinner			
	Bedtime			

NOTES:

Blood Sugar Tracker

WEEK OF: _______________

	Time	Before	After	Notes
	Breakfast			
	Lunch			
	Dinner			
	Bedtime			
	Breakfast			
	Lunch			
	Dinner			
	Bedtime			
	Breakfast			
	Lunch			
	Dinner			
	Bedtime			
	Breakfast			
	Lunch			
	Dinner			
	Bedtime			
	Breakfast			
	Lunch			
	Dinner			
	Bedtime			
	Breakfast			
	Lunch			
	Dinner			
	Bedtime			
	Breakfast			
	Lunch			
	Dinner			
	Bedtime			

Blood Sugar Tracker

WEEK OF: _________________

	Time	Before	After	Notes
Sunday	Breakfast Lunch Dinner Bedtime			
Monday	Breakfast Lunch Dinner Bedtime			
Tuesday	Breakfast Lunch Dinner Bedtime			
Wednesday	Breakfast Lunch Dinner Bedtime			
Thursday	Breakfast Lunch Dinner Bedtime			
Friday	Breakfast Lunch Dinner Bedtime			
Saturday	Breakfast Lunch Dinner Bedtime			

Blood Sugar Tracker

WEEK OF: _______________

	Time	Before	After	Notes
Sunday	Breakfast			
	Lunch			
	Dinner			
	Bedtime			
Monday	Breakfast			
	Lunch			
	Dinner			
	Bedtime			
Tuesday	Breakfast			
	Lunch			
	Dinner			
	Bedtime			
Wednesday	Breakfast			
	Lunch			
	Dinner			
	Bedtime			
Thursday	Breakfast			
	Lunch			
	Dinner			
	Bedtime			
Friday	Breakfast			
	Lunch			
	Dinner			
	Bedtime			
Saturday	Breakfast			
	Lunch			
	Dinner			
	Bedtime			

Blood Sugar Tracker

WEEK OF: ___________________

Sunday	Time	Before	After	Notes
	Breakfast			
	Lunch			
	Dinner			
	Bedtime			

Monday	Time	Before	After	Notes
	Breakfast			
	Lunch			
	Dinner			
	Bedtime			

Tuesday	Time	Before	After	Notes
	Breakfast			
	Lunch			
	Dinner			
	Bedtime			

Wednesday	Time	Before	After	Notes
	Breakfast			
	Lunch			
	Dinner			
	Bedtime			

Thursday	Time	Before	After	Notes
	Breakfast			
	Lunch			
	Dinner			
	Bedtime			

Friday	Time	Before	After	Notes
	Breakfast			
	Lunch			
	Dinner			
	Bedtime			

Saturday	Time	Before	After	Notes
	Breakfast			
	Lunch			
	Dinner			
	Bedtime			

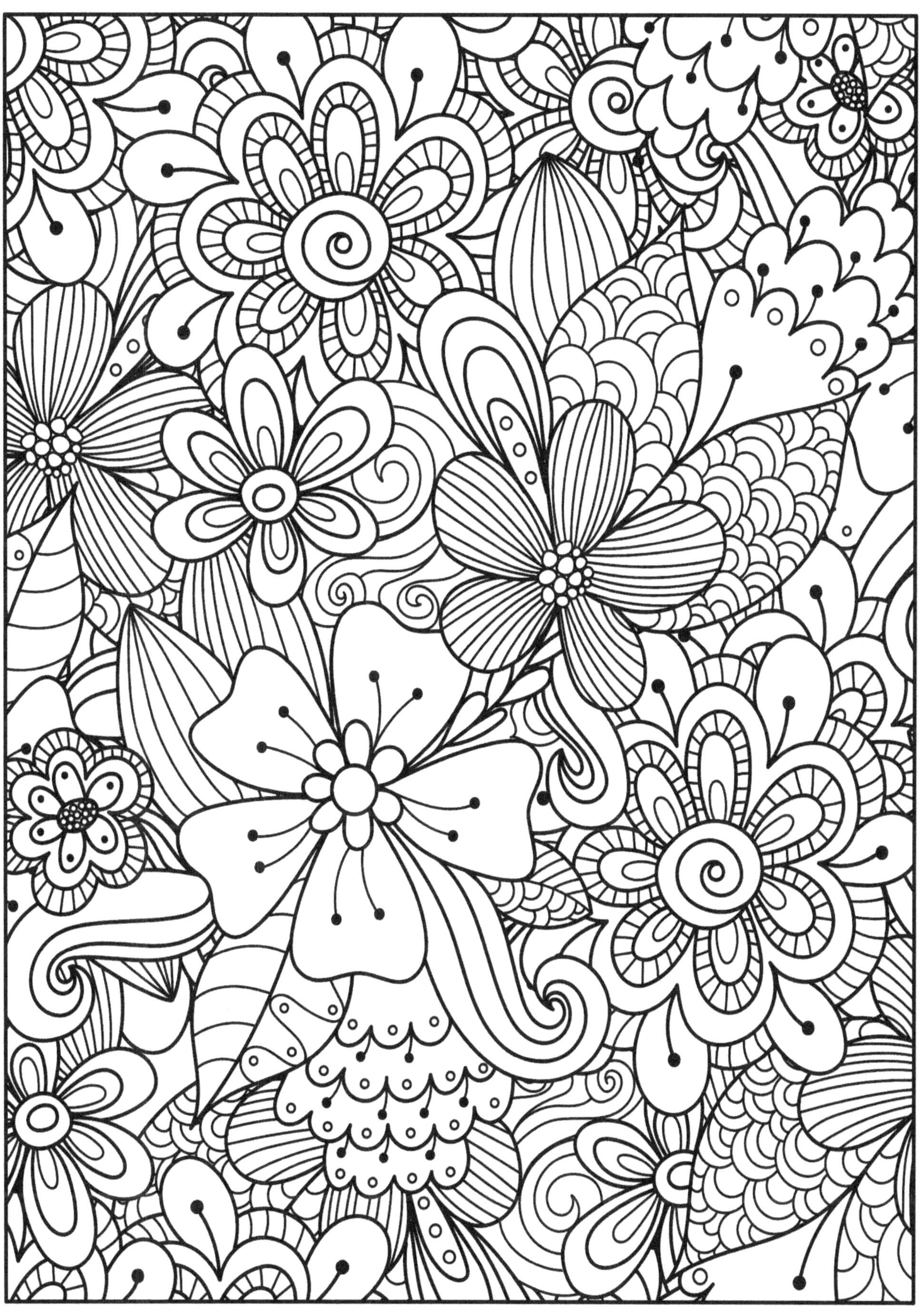

Blood Sugar Tracker

WEEK OF: _______________

Time	Before	After	Notes
Breakfast			
Lunch			
Dinner			
Bedtime			
Breakfast			
Lunch			
Dinner			
Bedtime			
Breakfast			
Lunch			
Dinner			
Bedtime			
Breakfast			
Lunch			
Dinner			
Bedtime			
Breakfast			
Lunch			
Dinner			
Bedtime			
Breakfast			
Lunch			
Dinner			
Bedtime			
Breakfast			
Lunch			
Dinner			
Bedtime			

Blood Sugar Tracker

WEEK OF: _______________

	Time	Before	After	Notes
Sunday	Breakfast			
	Lunch			
	Dinner			
	Bedtime			
Monday	Breakfast			
	Lunch			
	Dinner			
	Bedtime			
Tuesday	Breakfast			
	Lunch			
	Dinner			
	Bedtime			
Wednesday	Breakfast			
	Lunch			
	Dinner			
	Bedtime			
Thursday	Breakfast			
	Lunch			
	Dinner			
	Bedtime			
Friday	Breakfast			
	Lunch			
	Dinner			
	Bedtime			
Saturday	Breakfast			
	Lunch			
	Dinner			
	Bedtime			

Blood Sugar Tracker

WEEK OF: _________________

Time	Before	After	Notes
Breakfast			
Lunch			
Dinner			
Bedtime			
Breakfast			
Lunch			
Dinner			
Bedtime			
Breakfast			
Lunch			
Dinner			
Bedtime			
Breakfast			
Lunch			
Dinner			
Bedtime			
Breakfast			
Lunch			
Dinner			
Bedtime			
Breakfast			
Lunch			
Dinner			
Bedtime			
Breakfast			
Lunch			
Dinner			
Bedtime			

BLOOD SUGAR TRACKER

WEEK OF: _______________

	Time	Before	After	Notes
Sunday	BREAKFAST			
	LUNCH			
	DINNER			
	BEDTIME			
Monday	BREAKFAST			
	LUNCH			
	DINNER			
	BEDTIME			
Tuesday	BREAKFAST			
	LUNCH			
	DINNER			
	BEDTIME			
Wednesday	BREAKFAST			
	LUNCH			
	DINNER			
	BEDTIME			
Thursday	BREAKFAST			
	LUNCH			
	DINNER			
	BEDTIME			
Friday	BREAKFAST			
	LUNCH			
	DINNER			
	BEDTIME			
Saturday	BREAKFAST			
	LUNCH			
	DINNER			
	BEDTIME			

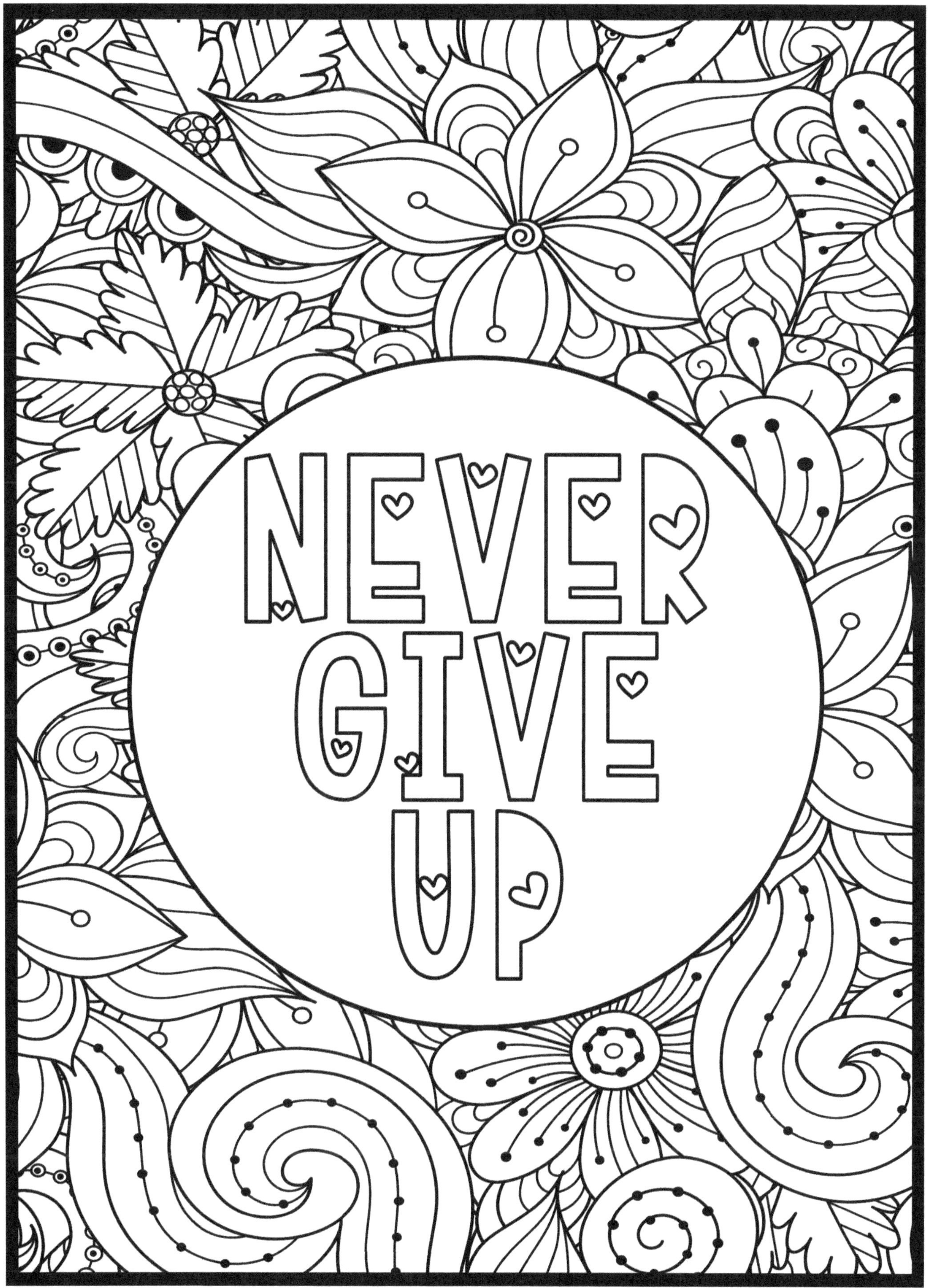

NEVER
GIVE
UP

Blood Sugar Tracker

WEEK OF: _________________

	Time	Before	After	Notes
Monday	Breakfast			
	Lunch			
	Dinner			
	Bedtime			
Tuesday	Breakfast			
	Lunch			
	Dinner			
	Bedtime			
Wednesday	Breakfast			
	Lunch			
	Dinner			
	Bedtime			
Thursday	Breakfast			
	Lunch			
	Dinner			
	Bedtime			
Friday	Breakfast			
	Lunch			
	Dinner			
	Bedtime			
Saturday	Breakfast			
	Lunch			
	Dinner			
	Bedtime			
Sunday	Breakfast			
	Lunch			
	Dinner			
	Bedtime			

Blood Sugar Tracker

WEEK OF: _______________________

	Time	Before	After	Notes
Sunday	Breakfast			
	Lunch			
	Dinner			
	Bedtime			
Monday	Breakfast			
	Lunch			
	Dinner			
	Bedtime			
Tuesday	Breakfast			
	Lunch			
	Dinner			
	Bedtime			
Wednesday	Breakfast			
	Lunch			
	Dinner			
	Bedtime			
Thursday	Breakfast			
	Lunch			
	Dinner			
	Bedtime			
Friday	Breakfast			
	Lunch			
	Dinner			
	Bedtime			
Saturday	Breakfast			
	Lunch			
	Dinner			
	Bedtime			

Blood Sugar Tracker

WEEK OF: ________________

Time	Before	After	Notes
Breakfast			
Lunch			
Dinner			
Bedtime			
Breakfast			
Lunch			
Dinner			
Bedtime			
Breakfast			
Lunch			
Dinner			
Bedtime			
Breakfast			
Lunch			
Dinner			
Bedtime			
Breakfast			
Lunch			
Dinner			
Bedtime			
Breakfast			
Lunch			
Dinner			
Bedtime			
Breakfast			
Lunch			
Dinner			
Bedtime			

Blood Sugar Tracker

	Time	Before	After	Notes
Sunday	Breakfast			
	Lunch			
	Dinner			
	Bedtime			
Monday	Breakfast			
	Lunch			
	Dinner			
	Bedtime			
Tuesday	Breakfast			
	Lunch			
	Dinner			
	Bedtime			
Wednesday	Breakfast			
	Lunch			
	Dinner			
	Bedtime			
Thursday	Breakfast			
	Lunch			
	Dinner			
	Bedtime			
Friday	Breakfast			
	Lunch			
	Dinner			
	Bedtime			
Saturday	Breakfast			
	Lunch			
	Dinner			
	Bedtime			

NOTES:

Blood Sugar Tracker

WEEK OF: _______________________

	Time	Before	After	Notes
Sunday	Breakfast			
	Lunch			
	Dinner			
	Bedtime			
Monday	Breakfast			
	Lunch			
	Dinner			
	Bedtime			
Tuesday	Breakfast			
	Lunch			
	Dinner			
	Bedtime			
Wednesday	Breakfast			
	Lunch			
	Dinner			
	Bedtime			
Thursday	Breakfast			
	Lunch			
	Dinner			
	Bedtime			
Friday	Breakfast			
	Lunch			
	Dinner			
	Bedtime			
Saturday	Breakfast			
	Lunch			
	Dinner			
	Bedtime			

Blood Sugar Tracker

WEEK OF: _________________

	Time	Before	After	Notes
Sunday	Breakfast			
	Lunch			
	Dinner			
	Bedtime			
Monday	Breakfast			
	Lunch			
	Dinner			
	Bedtime			
Tuesday	Breakfast			
	Lunch			
	Dinner			
	Bedtime			
Wednesday	Breakfast			
	Lunch			
	Dinner			
	Bedtime			
Thursday	Breakfast			
	Lunch			
	Dinner			
	Bedtime			
Friday	Breakfast			
	Lunch			
	Dinner			
	Bedtime			
Saturday	Breakfast			
	Lunch			
	Dinner			
	Bedtime			

Blood Sugar Tracker

WEEK OF: _______________

Sunday

- Breakfast
- Lunch
- Dinner
- Bedtime

Monday

- Breakfast
- Lunch
- Dinner
- Bedtime

Tuesday

- Breakfast
- Lunch
- Dinner
- Bedtime

Wednesday

- Breakfast
- Lunch
- Dinner
- Bedtime

Thursday

- Breakfast
- Lunch
- Dinner
- Bedtime

Friday

- Breakfast
- Lunch
- Dinner
- Bedtime

Saturday

- Breakfast
- Lunch
- Dinner
- Bedtime

Blood Sugar Tracker

WEEK OF: _________________

	Time	Before	After	Notes
Sunday	Breakfast			
	Lunch			
	Dinner			
	Bedtime			
Monday	Breakfast			
	Lunch			
	Dinner			
	Bedtime			
Tuesday	Breakfast			
	Lunch			
	Dinner			
	Bedtime			
Wednesday	Breakfast			
	Lunch			
	Dinner			
	Bedtime			
Thursday	Breakfast			
	Lunch			
	Dinner			
	Bedtime			
Friday	Breakfast			
	Lunch			
	Dinner			
	Bedtime			
Saturday	Breakfast			
	Lunch			
	Dinner			
	Bedtime			

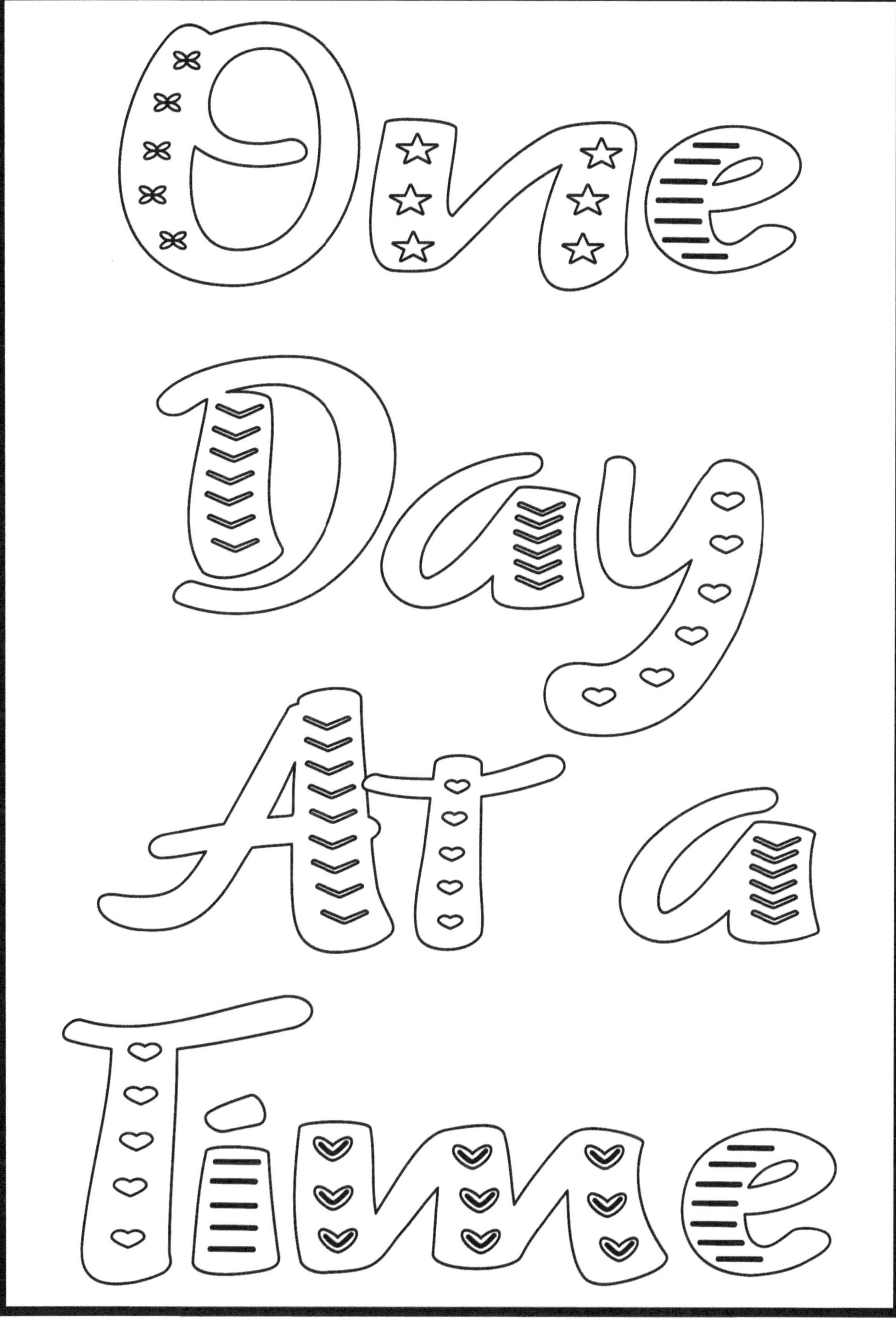

One
Day
At a
Time

Blood Sugar Tracker

WEEK OF: ___________________

	Time	Before	After	Notes
Sunday	Breakfast			
	Lunch			
	Dinner			
	Bedtime			
Monday	Breakfast			
	Lunch			
	Dinner			
	Bedtime			
Tuesday	Breakfast			
	Lunch			
	Dinner			
	Bedtime			
Wednesday	Breakfast			
	Lunch			
	Dinner			
	Bedtime			
Thursday	Breakfast			
	Lunch			
	Dinner			
	Bedtime			
Friday	Breakfast			
	Lunch			
	Dinner			
	Bedtime			
Saturday	Breakfast			
	Lunch			
	Dinner			
	Bedtime			

Blood Sugar Tracker

WEEK OF: _______________________

<table>
<tr><td rowspan="4"></td><td>Time</td><td>Before</td><td>After</td><td>Notes</td></tr>
</table>

	Time	Before	After	Notes
Sunday	Breakfast			
	Lunch			
	Dinner			
	Bedtime			
Monday	Breakfast			
	Lunch			
	Dinner			
	Bedtime			
Tuesday	Breakfast			
	Lunch			
	Dinner			
	Bedtime			
Wednesday	Breakfast			
	Lunch			
	Dinner			
	Bedtime			
Thursday	Breakfast			
	Lunch			
	Dinner			
	Bedtime			
Friday	Breakfast			
	Lunch			
	Dinner			
	Bedtime			
Saturday	Breakfast			
	Lunch			
	Dinner			
	Bedtime			

Blood Sugar Tracker

WEEK OF: _________________________

	Time	Before	After	Notes
Sunday	Breakfast Lunch Dinner Bedtime			
Monday	Breakfast Lunch Dinner Bedtime			
Tuesday	Breakfast Lunch Dinner Bedtime			
Wednesday	Breakfast Lunch Dinner Bedtime			
Thursday	Breakfast Lunch Dinner Bedtime			
Friday	Breakfast Lunch Dinner Bedtime			
Saturday	Breakfast Lunch Dinner Bedtime			

Blood Sugar Tracker

WEEK OF: _______________________

<table>
<tr><td rowspan="32">Saturday   Friday   Thursday   Wednesday   Tuesday   Monday   Sunday</td><td>Time</td><td>Before</td><td>After</td><td>Notes</td></tr>
<tr><td>Breakfast</td><td></td><td></td><td></td></tr>
<tr><td>Lunch</td><td></td><td></td><td></td></tr>
<tr><td>Dinner</td><td></td><td></td><td></td></tr>
<tr><td>Bedtime</td><td></td><td></td><td></td></tr>
<tr><td>Breakfast</td><td></td><td></td><td></td></tr>
<tr><td>Lunch</td><td></td><td></td><td></td></tr>
<tr><td>Dinner</td><td></td><td></td><td></td></tr>
<tr><td>Bedtime</td><td></td><td></td><td></td></tr>
<tr><td>Breakfast</td><td></td><td></td><td></td></tr>
<tr><td>Lunch</td><td></td><td></td><td></td></tr>
<tr><td>Dinner</td><td></td><td></td><td></td></tr>
<tr><td>Bedtime</td><td></td><td></td><td></td></tr>
<tr><td>Breakfast</td><td></td><td></td><td></td></tr>
<tr><td>Lunch</td><td></td><td></td><td></td></tr>
<tr><td>Dinner</td><td></td><td></td><td></td></tr>
<tr><td>Bedtime</td><td></td><td></td><td></td></tr>
<tr><td>Breakfast</td><td></td><td></td><td></td></tr>
<tr><td>Lunch</td><td></td><td></td><td></td></tr>
<tr><td>Dinner</td><td></td><td></td><td></td></tr>
<tr><td>Bedtime</td><td></td><td></td><td></td></tr>
<tr><td>Breakfast</td><td></td><td></td><td></td></tr>
<tr><td>Lunch</td><td></td><td></td><td></td></tr>
<tr><td>Dinner</td><td></td><td></td><td></td></tr>
<tr><td>Bedtime</td><td></td><td></td><td></td></tr>
<tr><td>Breakfast</td><td></td><td></td><td></td></tr>
<tr><td>Lunch</td><td></td><td></td><td></td></tr>
<tr><td>Dinner</td><td></td><td></td><td></td></tr>
<tr><td>Bedtime</td><td></td><td></td><td></td></tr>
</table>

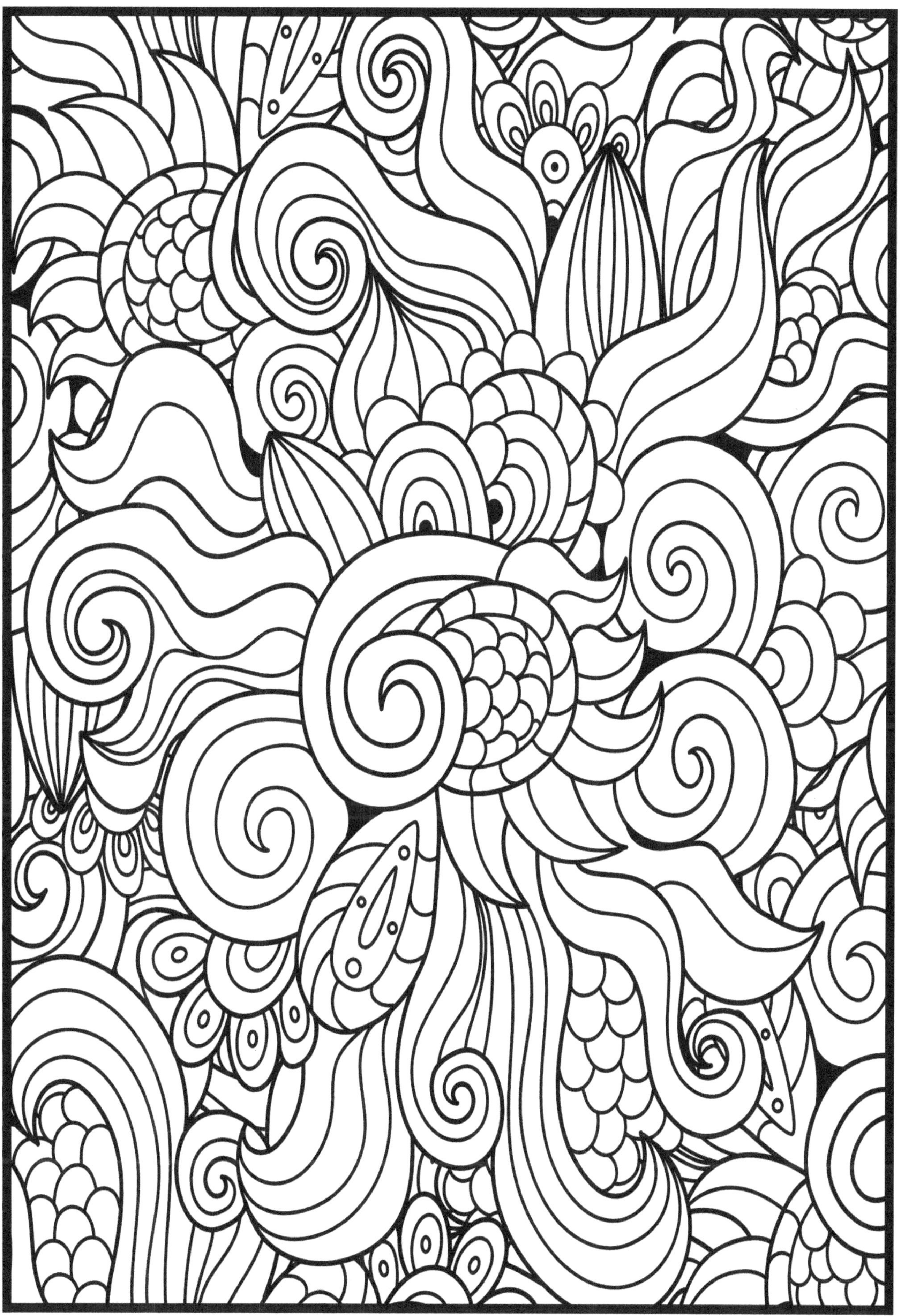

Blood Sugar Tracker

WEEK OF: _______________________

	Time	Before	After	Notes
Sunday	Breakfast			
	Lunch			
	Dinner			
	Bedtime			
Monday	Breakfast			
	Lunch			
	Dinner			
	Bedtime			
Tuesday	Breakfast			
	Lunch			
	Dinner			
	Bedtime			
Wednesday	Breakfast			
	Lunch			
	Dinner			
	Bedtime			
Thursday	Breakfast			
	Lunch			
	Dinner			
	Bedtime			
Friday	Breakfast			
	Lunch			
	Dinner			
	Bedtime			
Saturday	Breakfast			
	Lunch			
	Dinner			
	Bedtime			

Blood Sugar Tracker

WEEK OF: _________________

	Time	Before	After	Notes
Sunday	Breakfast Lunch Dinner Bedtime			
Monday	Breakfast Lunch Dinner Bedtime			
Tuesday	Breakfast Lunch Dinner Bedtime			
Wednesday	Breakfast Lunch Dinner Bedtime			
Thursday	Breakfast Lunch Dinner Bedtime			
Friday	Breakfast Lunch Dinner Bedtime			
Saturday	Breakfast Lunch Dinner Bedtime			

Blood Sugar Tracker

WEEK OF: _______________________

Time	Before	After	Notes
Breakfast			
Lunch			
Dinner			
Bedtime			
Breakfast			
Lunch			
Dinner			
Bedtime			
Breakfast			
Lunch			
Dinner			
Bedtime			
Breakfast			
Lunch			
Dinner			
Bedtime			
Breakfast			
Lunch			
Dinner			
Bedtime			
Breakfast			
Lunch			
Dinner			
Bedtime			
Breakfast			
Lunch			
Dinner			
Bedtime			

Blood Sugar Tracker

WEEK OF: _______________________

Time	Before	After	Notes
Breakfast			
Lunch			
Dinner			
Bedtime			
Breakfast			
Lunch			
Dinner			
Bedtime			
Breakfast			
Lunch			
Dinner			
Bedtime			
Breakfast			
Lunch			
Dinner			
Bedtime			
Breakfast			
Lunch			
Dinner			
Bedtime			
Breakfast			
Lunch			
Dinner			
Bedtime			
Breakfast			
Lunch			
Dinner			
Bedtime			

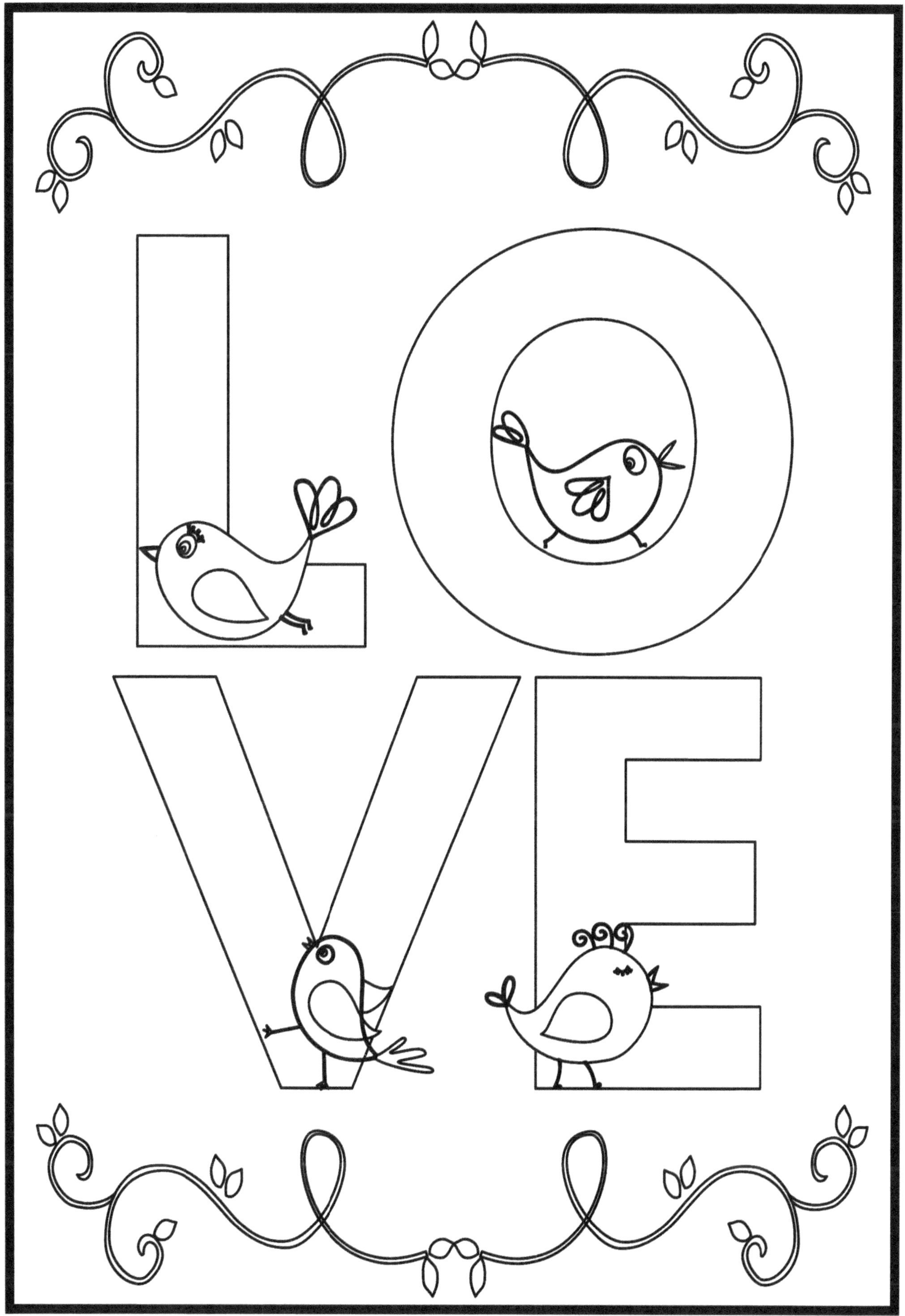

Blood Sugar Tracker

WEEK OF: _______________

Time	Before	After	Notes
Breakfast			
Lunch			
Dinner			
Bedtime			
Breakfast			
Lunch			
Dinner			
Bedtime			
Breakfast			
Lunch			
Dinner			
Bedtime			
Breakfast			
Lunch			
Dinner			
Bedtime			
Breakfast			
Lunch			
Dinner			
Bedtime			
Breakfast			
Lunch			
Dinner			
Bedtime			
Breakfast			
Lunch			
Dinner			
Bedtime			

Blood Sugar Tracker

WEEK OF: _________________

	Time	Before	After	Notes
Sunday	Breakfast			
	Lunch			
	Dinner			
	Bedtime			
Monday	Breakfast			
	Lunch			
	Dinner			
	Bedtime			
Tuesday	Breakfast			
	Lunch			
	Dinner			
	Bedtime			
Wednesday	Breakfast			
	Lunch			
	Dinner			
	Bedtime			
Thursday	Breakfast			
	Lunch			
	Dinner			
	Bedtime			
Friday	Breakfast			
	Lunch			
	Dinner			
	Bedtime			
Saturday	Breakfast			
	Lunch			
	Dinner			
	Bedtime			

Blood Sugar Tracker

WEEK OF: _______________________

	Time	Before	After	Notes
Monday	Breakfast			
	Lunch			
	Dinner			
	Bedtime			
Tuesday	Breakfast			
	Lunch			
	Dinner			
	Bedtime			
Wednesday	Breakfast			
	Lunch			
	Dinner			
	Bedtime			
Thursday	Breakfast			
	Lunch			
	Dinner			
	Bedtime			
Friday	Breakfast			
	Lunch			
	Dinner			
	Bedtime			
Saturday	Breakfast			
	Lunch			
	Dinner			
	Bedtime			
Sunday	Breakfast			
	Lunch			
	Dinner			
	Bedtime			

Blood Sugar Tracker

WEEK OF: _______________________

	Time	Before	After	Notes
Sunday	Breakfast Lunch Dinner Bedtime			
Monday	Breakfast Lunch Dinner Bedtime			
Tuesday	Breakfast Lunch Dinner Bedtime			
Wednesday	Breakfast Lunch Dinner Bedtime			
Thursday	Breakfast Lunch Dinner Bedtime			
Friday	Breakfast Lunch Dinner Bedtime			
Saturday	Breakfast Lunch Dinner Bedtime			

NOTES:

Blood Sugar Tracker

WEEK OF: ______________________

<table>
<tr><th></th><th>Time</th><th>Before</th><th>After</th><th>Notes</th></tr>
<tr><td rowspan="4">Sunday</td><td>Breakfast</td><td></td><td></td><td></td></tr>
<tr><td>Lunch</td><td></td><td></td><td></td></tr>
<tr><td>Dinner</td><td></td><td></td><td></td></tr>
<tr><td>Bedtime</td><td></td><td></td><td></td></tr>
<tr><td rowspan="4">Monday</td><td>Breakfast</td><td></td><td></td><td></td></tr>
<tr><td>Lunch</td><td></td><td></td><td></td></tr>
<tr><td>Dinner</td><td></td><td></td><td></td></tr>
<tr><td>Bedtime</td><td></td><td></td><td></td></tr>
<tr><td rowspan="4">Tuesday</td><td>Breakfast</td><td></td><td></td><td></td></tr>
<tr><td>Lunch</td><td></td><td></td><td></td></tr>
<tr><td>Dinner</td><td></td><td></td><td></td></tr>
<tr><td>Bedtime</td><td></td><td></td><td></td></tr>
<tr><td rowspan="4">Wednesday</td><td>Breakfast</td><td></td><td></td><td></td></tr>
<tr><td>Lunch</td><td></td><td></td><td></td></tr>
<tr><td>Dinner</td><td></td><td></td><td></td></tr>
<tr><td>Bedtime</td><td></td><td></td><td></td></tr>
<tr><td rowspan="4">Thursday</td><td>Breakfast</td><td></td><td></td><td></td></tr>
<tr><td>Lunch</td><td></td><td></td><td></td></tr>
<tr><td>Dinner</td><td></td><td></td><td></td></tr>
<tr><td>Bedtime</td><td></td><td></td><td></td></tr>
<tr><td rowspan="4">Friday</td><td>Breakfast</td><td></td><td></td><td></td></tr>
<tr><td>Lunch</td><td></td><td></td><td></td></tr>
<tr><td>Dinner</td><td></td><td></td><td></td></tr>
<tr><td>Bedtime</td><td></td><td></td><td></td></tr>
<tr><td rowspan="4">Saturday</td><td>Breakfast</td><td></td><td></td><td></td></tr>
<tr><td>Lunch</td><td></td><td></td><td></td></tr>
<tr><td>Dinner</td><td></td><td></td><td></td></tr>
<tr><td>Bedtime</td><td></td><td></td><td></td></tr>
</table>

Blood Sugar Tracker

WEEK OF: _________________

	Time	Before	After	Notes
Sunday	Breakfast			
	Lunch			
	Dinner			
	Bedtime			
Monday	Breakfast			
	Lunch			
	Dinner			
	Bedtime			
Tuesday	Breakfast			
	Lunch			
	Dinner			
	Bedtime			
Wednesday	Breakfast			
	Lunch			
	Dinner			
	Bedtime			
Thursday	Breakfast			
	Lunch			
	Dinner			
	Bedtime			
Friday	Breakfast			
	Lunch			
	Dinner			
	Bedtime			
Saturday	Breakfast			
	Lunch			
	Dinner			
	Bedtime			

Blood Sugar Tracker

WEEK OF: _______________

Time	Before	After	Notes
Breakfast			
Lunch			
Dinner			
Bedtime			
Breakfast			
Lunch			
Dinner			
Bedtime			
Breakfast			
Lunch			
Dinner			
Bedtime			
Breakfast			
Lunch			
Dinner			
Bedtime			
Breakfast			
Lunch			
Dinner			
Bedtime			
Breakfast			
Lunch			
Dinner			
Bedtime			
Breakfast			
Lunch			
Dinner			
Bedtime			

Blood Sugar Tracker

WEEK OF: _______________________

	Time	Before	After	Notes
Sunday	Breakfast			
	Lunch			
	Dinner			
	Bedtime			
Monday	Breakfast			
	Lunch			
	Dinner			
	Bedtime			
Tuesday	Breakfast			
	Lunch			
	Dinner			
	Bedtime			
Wednesday	Breakfast			
	Lunch			
	Dinner			
	Bedtime			
Thursday	Breakfast			
	Lunch			
	Dinner			
	Bedtime			
Friday	Breakfast			
	Lunch			
	Dinner			
	Bedtime			
Saturday	Breakfast			
	Lunch			
	Dinner			
	Bedtime			

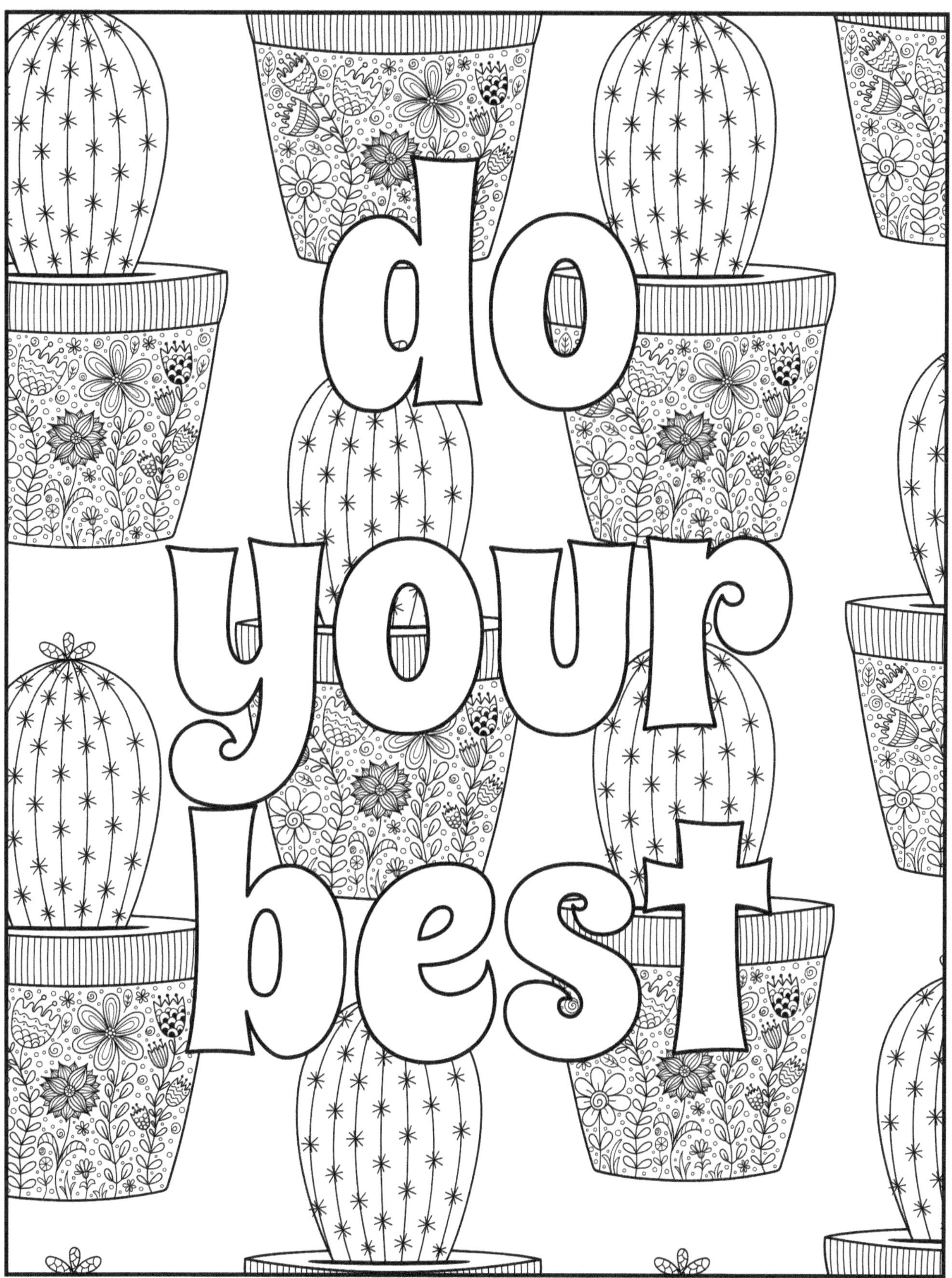

do
your
best

Blood Sugar Tracker

WEEK OF: _______________________

	Time	Before	After	Notes
	Breakfast			
	Lunch			
	Dinner			
	Bedtime			
	Breakfast			
	Lunch			
	Dinner			
	Bedtime			
	Breakfast			
	Lunch			
	Dinner			
	Bedtime			
	Breakfast			
	Lunch			
	Dinner			
	Bedtime			
	Breakfast			
	Lunch			
	Dinner			
	Bedtime			
	Breakfast			
	Lunch			
	Dinner			
	Bedtime			
	Breakfast			
	Lunch			
	Dinner			
	Bedtime			

Blood Sugar Tracker

WEEK OF: _________________

Time	Before	After	Notes
Breakfast			
Lunch			
Dinner			
Bedtime			
Breakfast			
Lunch			
Dinner			
Bedtime			
Breakfast			
Lunch			
Dinner			
Bedtime			
Breakfast			
Lunch			
Dinner			
Bedtime			
Breakfast			
Lunch			
Dinner			
Bedtime			
Breakfast			
Lunch			
Dinner			
Bedtime			
Breakfast			
Lunch			
Dinner			
Bedtime			

Blood Sugar Tracker

WEEK OF: _______________

	Time	Before	After	Notes
Sunday	Breakfast Lunch Dinner Bedtime			
Monday	Breakfast Lunch Dinner Bedtime			
Tuesday	Breakfast Lunch Dinner Bedtime			
Wednesday	Breakfast Lunch Dinner Bedtime			
Thursday	Breakfast Lunch Dinner Bedtime			
Friday	Breakfast Lunch Dinner Bedtime			
Saturday	Breakfast Lunch Dinner Bedtime			

Blood Sugar Tracker

WEEK OF: _______________________

	Time	Before	After	Notes
Sunday	Breakfast			
	Lunch			
	Dinner			
	Bedtime			
Monday	Breakfast			
	Lunch			
	Dinner			
	Bedtime			
Tuesday	Breakfast			
	Lunch			
	Dinner			
	Bedtime			
Wednesday	Breakfast			
	Lunch			
	Dinner			
	Bedtime			
Thursday	Breakfast			
	Lunch			
	Dinner			
	Bedtime			
Friday	Breakfast			
	Lunch			
	Dinner			
	Bedtime			
Saturday	Breakfast			
	Lunch			
	Dinner			
	Bedtime			

NOTES:

Blood Sugar Tracker

WEEK OF: _____________________

	Time	Before	After	Notes
	Breakfast			
	Lunch			
	Dinner			
	Bedtime			
	Breakfast			
	Lunch			
	Dinner			
	Bedtime			
	Breakfast			
	Lunch			
	Dinner			
	Bedtime			
	Breakfast			
	Lunch			
	Dinner			
	Bedtime			
	Breakfast			
	Lunch			
	Dinner			
	Bedtime			
	Breakfast			
	Lunch			
	Dinner			
	Bedtime			
	Breakfast			
	Lunch			
	Dinner			
	Bedtime			

Blood Sugar Tracker

WEEK OF: ___________________

	Time	Before	After	Notes
Sunday	Breakfast			
	Lunch			
	Dinner			
	Bedtime			
Monday	Breakfast			
	Lunch			
	Dinner			
	Bedtime			
Tuesday	Breakfast			
	Lunch			
	Dinner			
	Bedtime			
Wednesday	Breakfast			
	Lunch			
	Dinner			
	Bedtime			
Thursday	Breakfast			
	Lunch			
	Dinner			
	Bedtime			
Friday	Breakfast			
	Lunch			
	Dinner			
	Bedtime			
Saturday	Breakfast			
	Lunch			
	Dinner			
	Bedtime			

Blood Sugar Tracker

WEEK OF: _________________

	Time	Before	After	Notes
Sunday	Breakfast			
	Lunch			
	Dinner			
	Bedtime			
Monday	Breakfast			
	Lunch			
	Dinner			
	Bedtime			
Tuesday	Breakfast			
	Lunch			
	Dinner			
	Bedtime			
Wednesday	Breakfast			
	Lunch			
	Dinner			
	Bedtime			
Thursday	Breakfast			
	Lunch			
	Dinner			
	Bedtime			
Friday	Breakfast			
	Lunch			
	Dinner			
	Bedtime			
Saturday	Breakfast			
	Lunch			
	Dinner			
	Bedtime			

Blood Sugar Tracker

WEEK OF: ________________________

Sunday	Time	Before	After	Notes
	Breakfast			
	Lunch			
	Dinner			
	Bedtime			

Monday	Time	Before	After	Notes
	Breakfast			
	Lunch			
	Dinner			
	Bedtime			

Tuesday	Time	Before	After	Notes
	Breakfast			
	Lunch			
	Dinner			
	Bedtime			

Wednesday	Time	Before	After	Notes
	Breakfast			
	Lunch			
	Dinner			
	Bedtime			

Thursday	Time	Before	After	Notes
	Breakfast			
	Lunch			
	Dinner			
	Bedtime			

Friday	Time	Before	After	Notes
	Breakfast			
	Lunch			
	Dinner			
	Bedtime			

Saturday	Time	Before	After	Notes
	Breakfast			
	Lunch			
	Dinner			
	Bedtime			

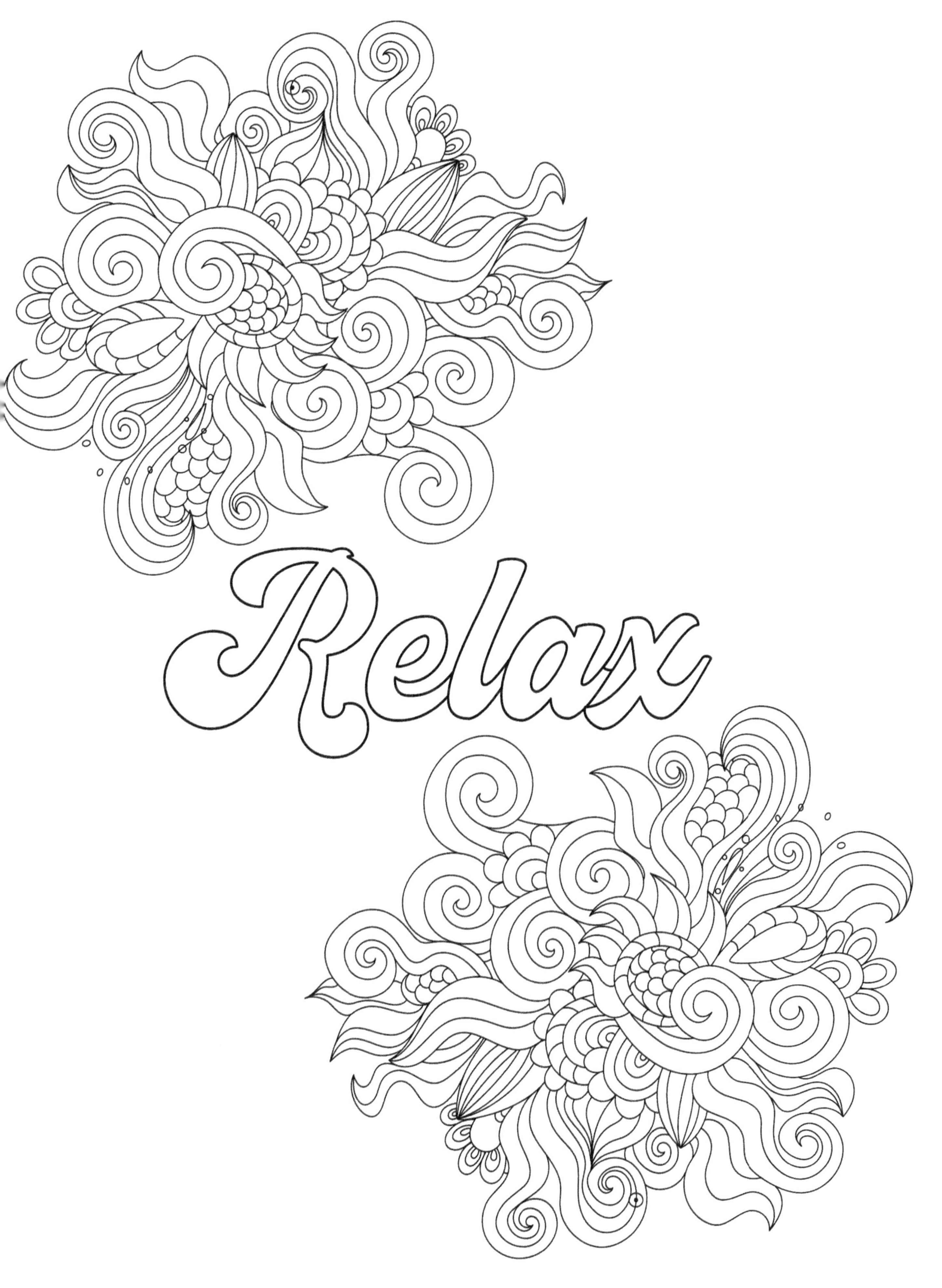
Relax

Blood Sugar Tracker

WEEK OF: _________________

	Time	Before	After	Notes
Sunday	Breakfast Lunch Dinner Bedtime			
Monday	Breakfast Lunch Dinner Bedtime			
Tuesday	Breakfast Lunch Dinner Bedtime			
Wednesday	Breakfast Lunch Dinner Bedtime			
Thursday	Breakfast Lunch Dinner Bedtime			
Friday	Breakfast Lunch Dinner Bedtime			
Saturday	Breakfast Lunch Dinner Bedtime			

Blood Sugar Tracker

WEEK OF: ________________

	Time	Before	After	Notes
Sunday	Breakfast			
	Lunch			
	Dinner			
	Bedtime			
Monday	Breakfast			
	Lunch			
	Dinner			
	Bedtime			
Tuesday	Breakfast			
	Lunch			
	Dinner			
	Bedtime			
Wednesday	Breakfast			
	Lunch			
	Dinner			
	Bedtime			
Thursday	Breakfast			
	Lunch			
	Dinner			
	Bedtime			
Friday	Breakfast			
	Lunch			
	Dinner			
	Bedtime			
Saturday	Breakfast			
	Lunch			
	Dinner			
	Bedtime			

Blood Sugar Tracker

WEEK OF: _______________

	Time	Before	After	Notes
Sunday	Breakfast			
	Lunch			
	Dinner			
	Bedtime			
Monday	Breakfast			
	Lunch			
	Dinner			
	Bedtime			
Tuesday	Breakfast			
	Lunch			
	Dinner			
	Bedtime			
Wednesday	Breakfast			
	Lunch			
	Dinner			
	Bedtime			
Thursday	Breakfast			
	Lunch			
	Dinner			
	Bedtime			
Friday	Breakfast			
	Lunch			
	Dinner			
	Bedtime			
Saturday	Breakfast			
	Lunch			
	Dinner			
	Bedtime			

Blood Sugar Tracker

WEEK OF: _________________

	Time	Before	After	Notes
Sunday	Breakfast Lunch Dinner Bedtime			
Monday	Breakfast Lunch Dinner Bedtime			
Tuesday	Breakfast Lunch Dinner Bedtime			
Wednesday	Breakfast Lunch Dinner Bedtime			
Thursday	Breakfast Lunch Dinner Bedtime			
Friday	Breakfast Lunch Dinner Bedtime			
Saturday	Breakfast Lunch Dinner Bedtime			

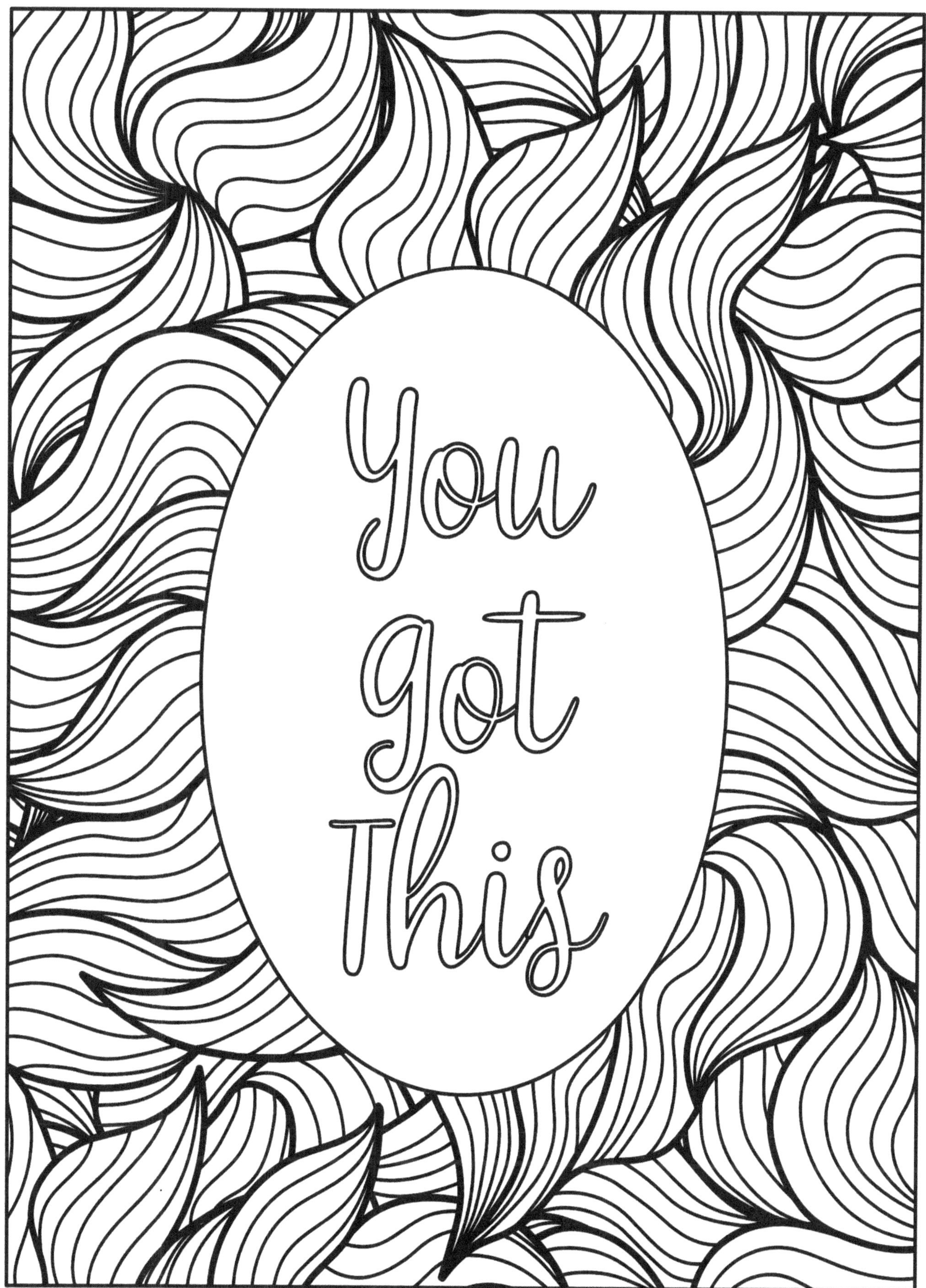

You got This

Blood Sugar Tracker

WEEK OF: _______________

	Time	Before	After	Notes
Sunday	Breakfast			
	Lunch			
	Dinner			
	Bedtime			
Monday	Breakfast			
	Lunch			
	Dinner			
	Bedtime			
Tuesday	Breakfast			
	Lunch			
	Dinner			
	Bedtime			
Wednesday	Breakfast			
	Lunch			
	Dinner			
	Bedtime			
Thursday	Breakfast			
	Lunch			
	Dinner			
	Bedtime			
Friday	Breakfast			
	Lunch			
	Dinner			
	Bedtime			
Saturday	Breakfast			
	Lunch			
	Dinner			
	Bedtime			

Blood Sugar Tracker

WEEK OF: ___________________

Sunday	Time	Before	After	Notes
	Breakfast			
	Lunch			
	Dinner			
	Bedtime			

Monday	Time	Before	After	Notes
	Breakfast			
	Lunch			
	Dinner			
	Bedtime			

Tuesday	Time	Before	After	Notes
	Breakfast			
	Lunch			
	Dinner			
	Bedtime			

Wednesday	Time	Before	After	Notes
	Breakfast			
	Lunch			
	Dinner			
	Bedtime			

Thursday	Time	Before	After	Notes
	Breakfast			
	Lunch			
	Dinner			
	Bedtime			

Friday	Time	Before	After	Notes
	Breakfast			
	Lunch			
	Dinner			
	Bedtime			

Saturday	Time	Before	After	Notes
	Breakfast			
	Lunch			
	Dinner			
	Bedtime			

Blood Sugar Tracker

WEEK OF: _______________________

	Time	Before	After	Notes
Sunday	Breakfast			
	Lunch			
	Dinner			
	Bedtime			
Monday	Breakfast			
	Lunch			
	Dinner			
	Bedtime			
Tuesday	Breakfast			
	Lunch			
	Dinner			
	Bedtime			
Wednesday	Breakfast			
	Lunch			
	Dinner			
	Bedtime			
Thursday	Breakfast			
	Lunch			
	Dinner			
	Bedtime			
Friday	Breakfast			
	Lunch			
	Dinner			
	Bedtime			
Saturday	Breakfast			
	Lunch			
	Dinner			
	Bedtime			

Blood Sugar Tracker

WEEK OF: _____________________

	Time	Before	After	Notes
Sunday	Breakfast Lunch Dinner Bedtime			
Monday	Breakfast Lunch Dinner Bedtime			
Tuesday	Breakfast Lunch Dinner Bedtime			
Wednesday	Breakfast Lunch Dinner Bedtime			
Thursday	Breakfast Lunch Dinner Bedtime			
Friday	Breakfast Lunch Dinner Bedtime			
Saturday	Breakfast Lunch Dinner Bedtime			

NOTES: